Emily's Allergy

Betty Forhman
Lyn Hochhauser,
Illustrator

Emily's Allergy

Forward:

The allergic child lives in a hostile ocean of her or his everyday environment. Surrounded by the normal things that we all touch — and inhale — and eat, she is besieged by uncomfortable nasal symptoms, eye symptoms, wheezing or hives.

This little book portrays one little girl's unhappiness at being separated from a friend. Frequently, this is the child's major motive for seeking help from an allergist. From a more realistic point of view, however, it is the unrelenting commonplace exposure — to grass pollen, to house dust, or mold spores or milk — which is little Emily's major problem.

It is the allergist's job to search the child's entire problem according to its relieve importance. He must be part botanist, part immunologist, sometimes father figure, at other time confidant, gourmet, weather profit, expert on the pharmacology of drugs and mechanically adept at handling the instruments of his profession.

When all is said and done, he is little Emily's affectionate friend and ally in her fight for normalcy.

Donald K Adler, M.D.
Former Chief, Pediatric Allergy
Mount Sinai Hospital
New York, New York

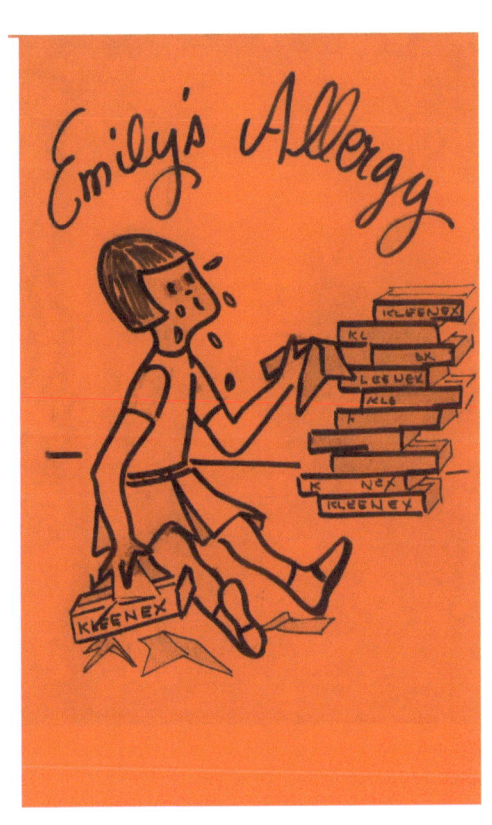

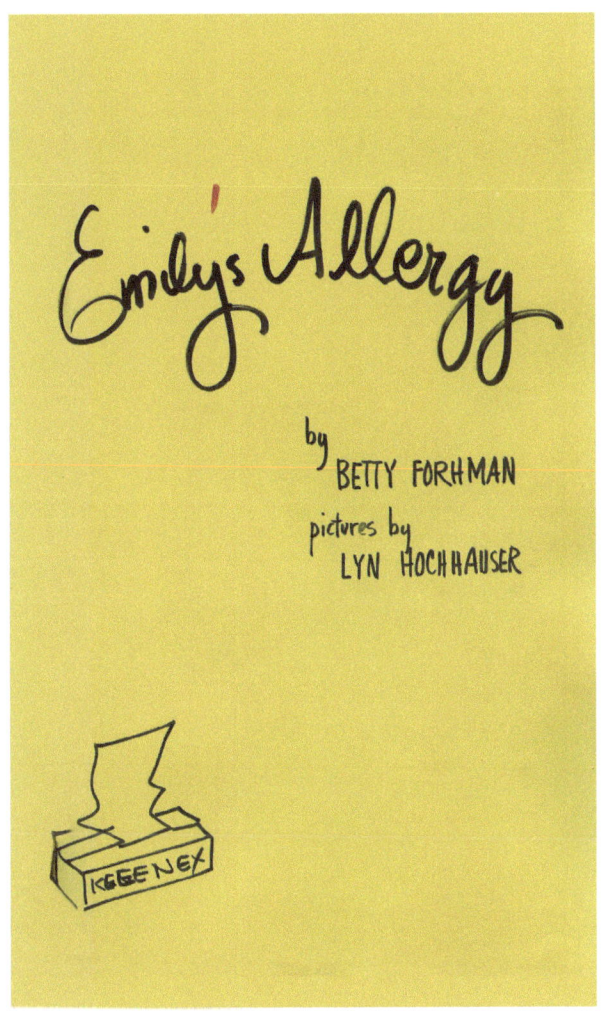

Emily's Allergy

by BETTY FORHMAN

pictures by
LYN HOCHHAUSER

ONCE
THERE
WAS
A
GIRL
NAMED EMILY
WHO
ADORED
CATS

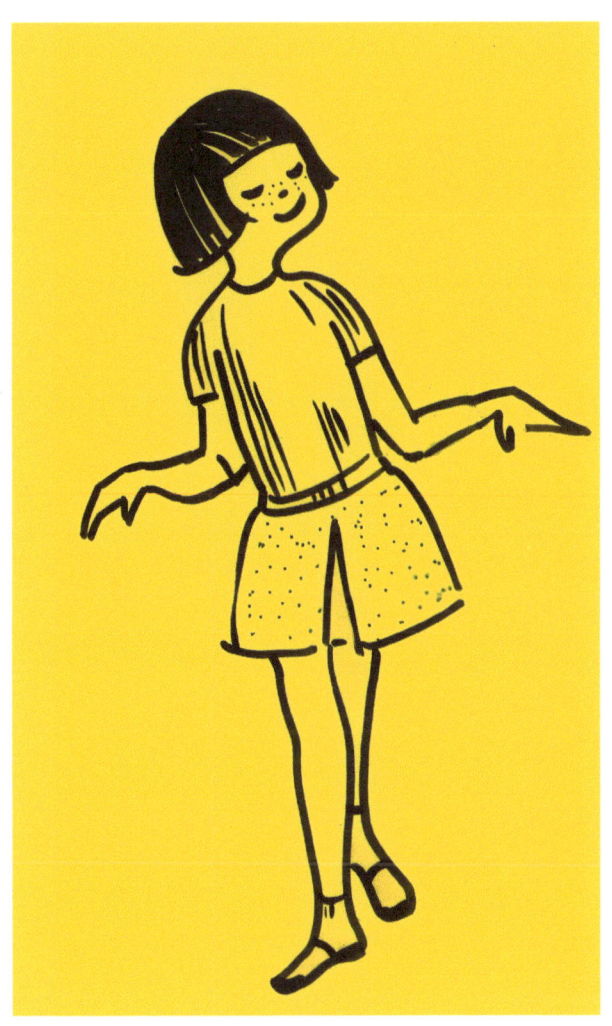

SHE LOVED
THEIR SOFT
FURRINESS,
THEIR FURRINESS
AND THE
CUDDLING WAY
THEY RUSHED
UP AGAINST
HER LEGS.

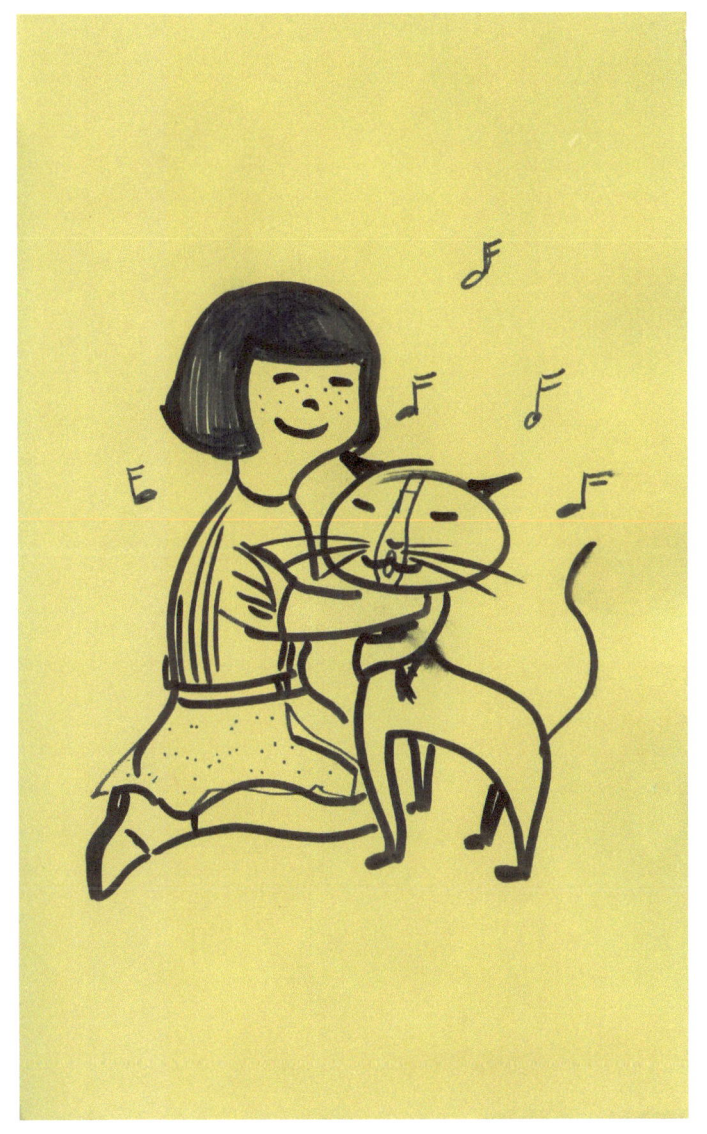

EMILY
OFTEN
WISHED
SHE
COULD
HAVE
A
CAT
OF
HER
OWN.
BUT
SHE
COULDN'T!

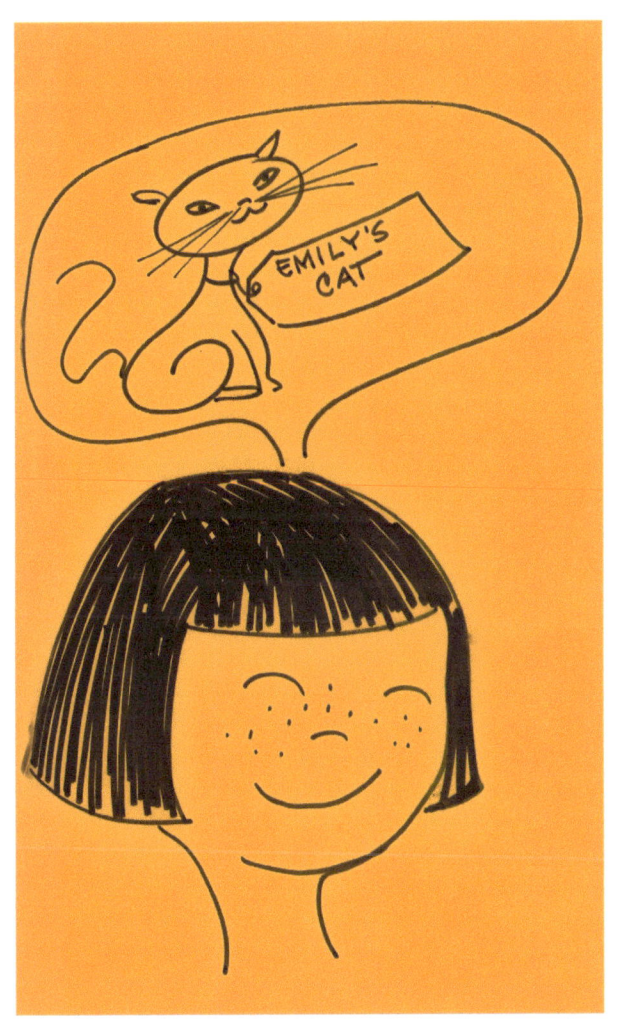

BECAUSE
EVERY
TIME
EMILY
PETTED
A
CAT,

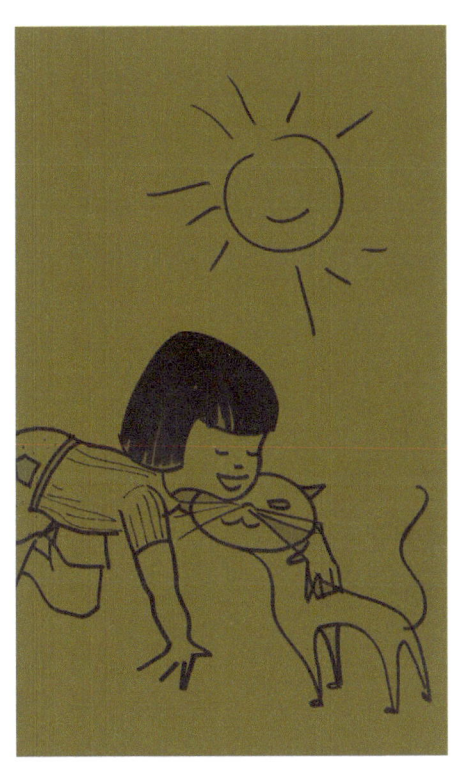

SHE
SNEEZED
AND
SNEEZED!
HER
EYES
GREW
RED
AND
REDDER!

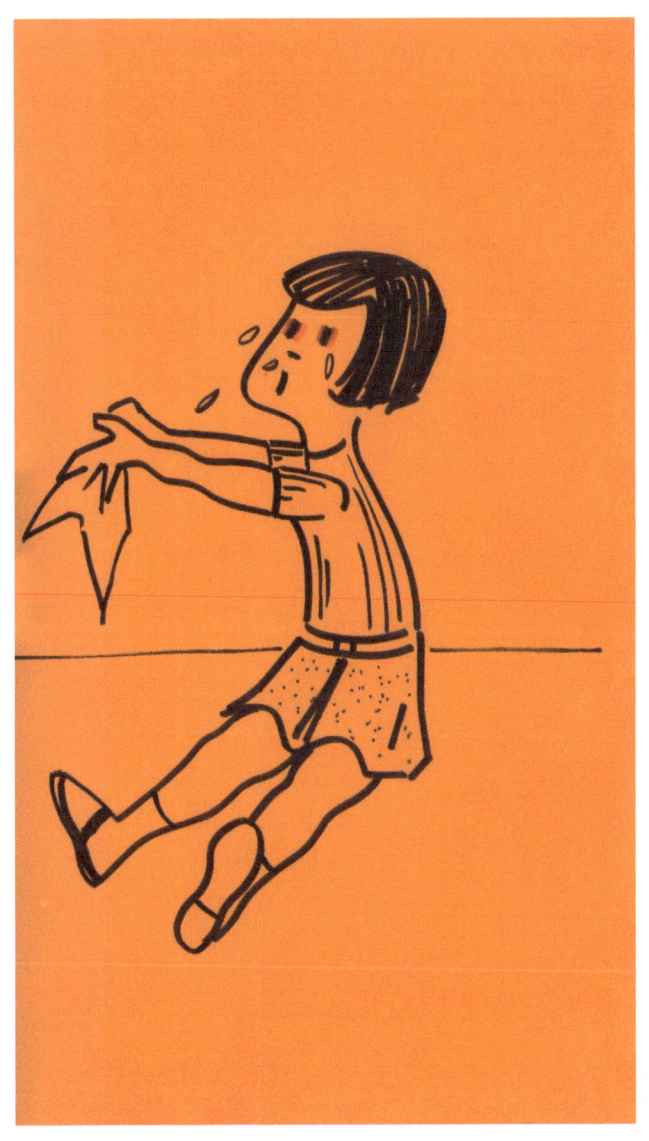

SHE
USED
MILLIONS
OF
TISSUES
AND
BILLIONS
OF
TISSUES
AND
TRILLIONS
OF
TISSUES!

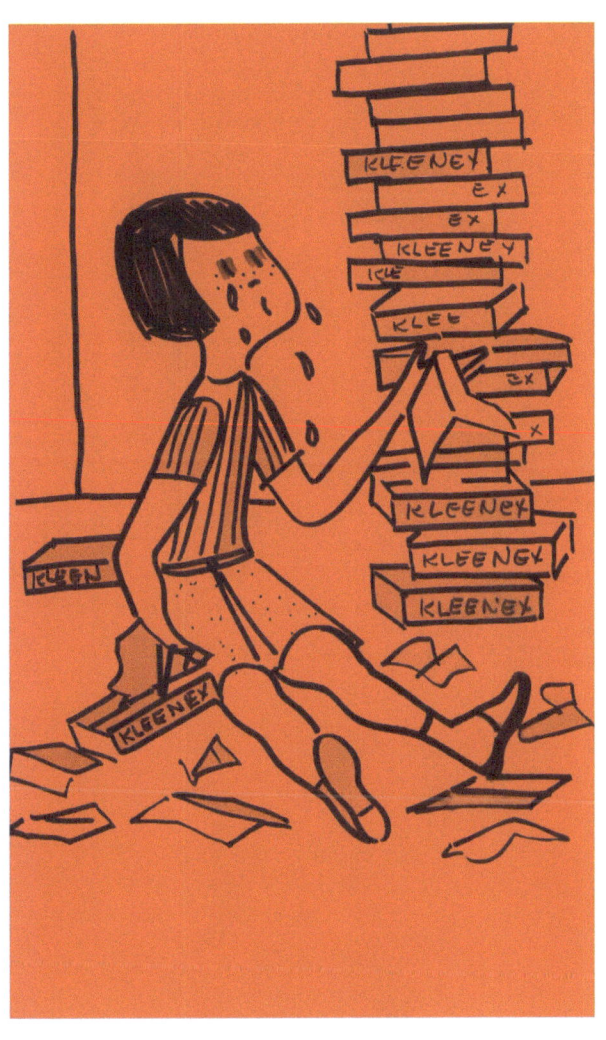

HER MOTHER SAID,
"EMILY, HONEY
DON'T PET ANY
CATS.
WHEN YOU DO,
YOU SNEEZE
AND WHEEZE
AND YOU USE UP
ALL THE TISSUES
WE HAVE."
EMILY SAID,
"I PROMISE
NOT TO PET CATS.
I WILL ONLY TALK
TO THEM."

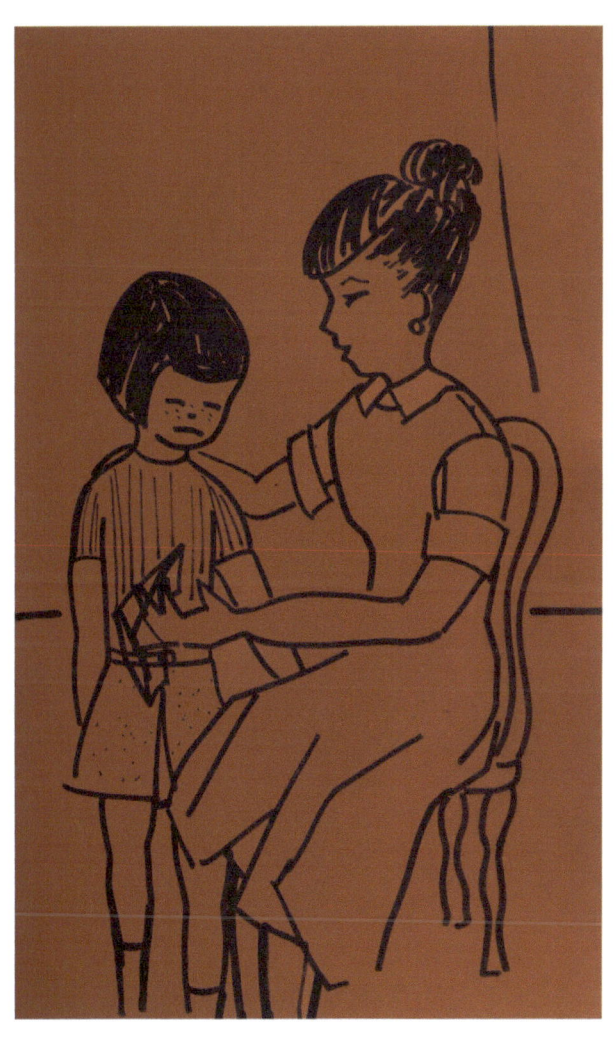

EMILY
WANTED
TO
RETURN
THE GREETING…
BY
PETTING THE CAT
MINNIE'S HEAD…
BUT
SHE COULDN'T!
SHE
HAD
PROMISED!

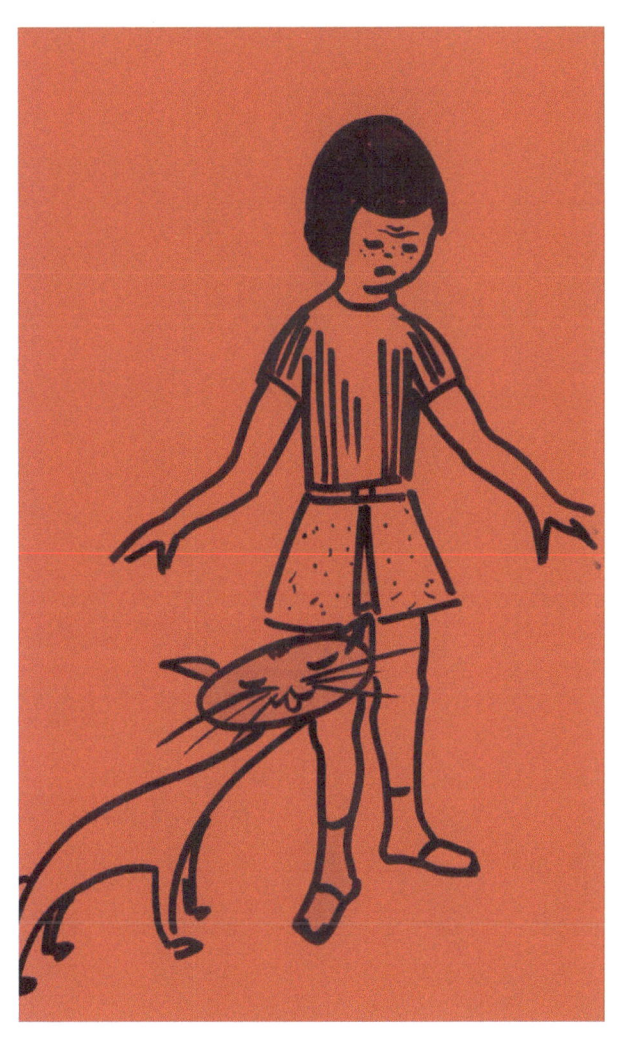

EMILY SAID,
"MINNIE, I STILL
LOVE YOU.
BUT WHENEVER I
PET YOU,
I SNEEZE AND WHEEZE.
MY EYES GROW
RED AND REDDER
AND I USE
TRILLIONS OF TISSUES.
MINNIE SEEMED
INTERESTED
AND EMILY PLEADED,
"MINNIE, LET'S BE
TALKING FRIENDS
INSTEAD OF
TOUCHING FRIENDS,
O.K.?"

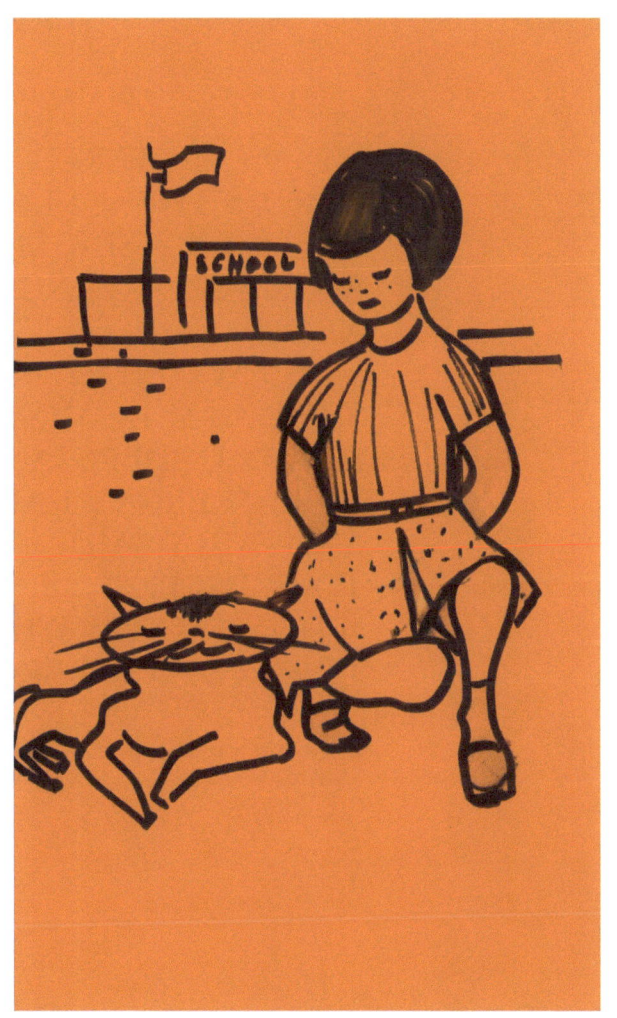

MINNIE PATTERED
ACROSS THE STREET
WITHOUT A SINGLE
BACKWARD GLANCE
AT EMILY.
EMILY WAS VERY SAD.
SHE WAS SURE MINNIE
DIDN'T UNDERSTAND
HER ALLERGY AT ALL!
AND EMILY SAID
TO HERSELF,
"I DON'T KNOW WHY I HAVE
TO HAVE AN ALLERGY
EITHER.
IT'S NOT FAIR!"

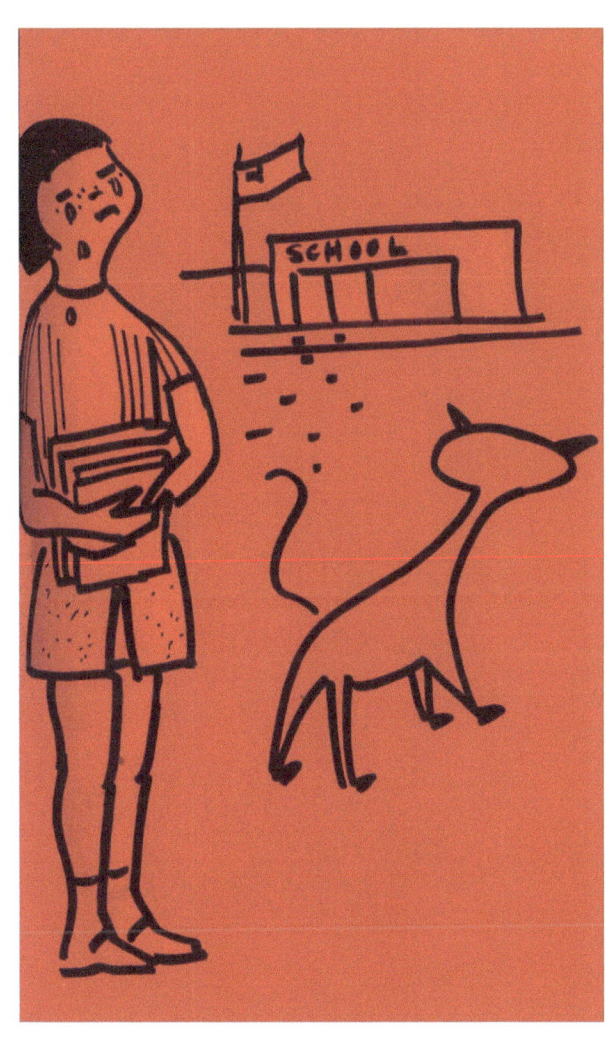

WHEN EMILY
CAME HOME
FROM SCHOOL,
SHE TOLD
HER MOTHER
ABOUT MEETING MINNIE
AND HOW MINNIE
DIDN'T UNDERSTAND.
EMILY SAID, "MOMMY, I
FEEL SAD ALL OVER!"
EMILY'S MOTHER NODDED
AND SAID, "I KNOW HOW
YOU FEEL.. THAT'S WHY
I JUST CALLED DR. ADLER
FOR AN APPOINTMENT. HE'S
A SPECIAL KIND OF
DOCTOR,
AN ALLERGIST."

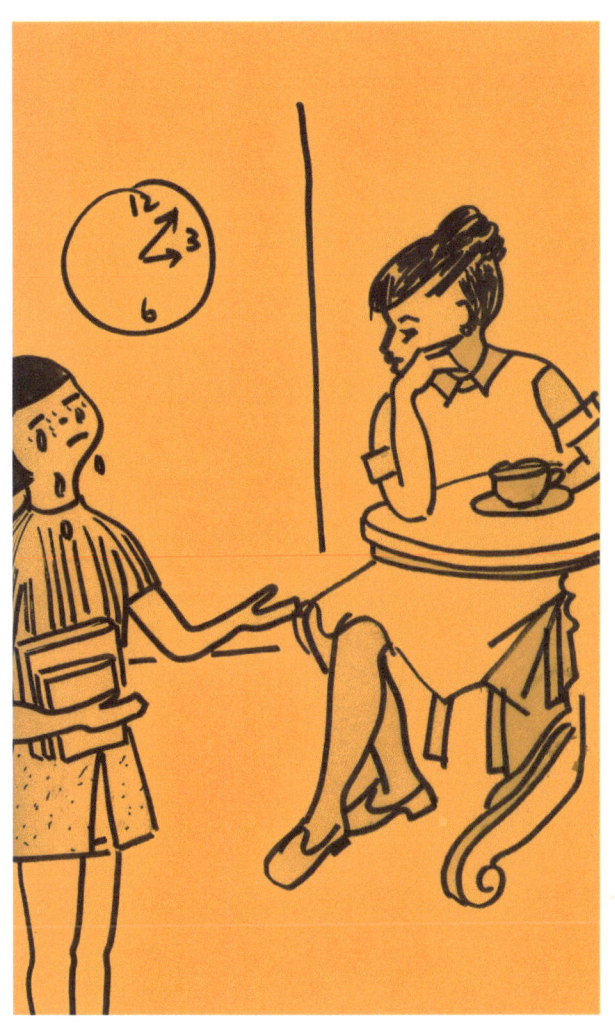

"THERE ARE MANY
CHILDREN
JUST LIKE YOU
WITH ALLERGIES.
DR. ADLER TAKES SPECIAL
MEDICINE AND INJECTS
THE SKIN ON CHILDREN'S
ARMS AND MAKES THEIR
ALLERGIES DISAPPEAR
EVENTUALLY." EMILY'S
EYES GREW W-I-D-E
WITH WONDER.

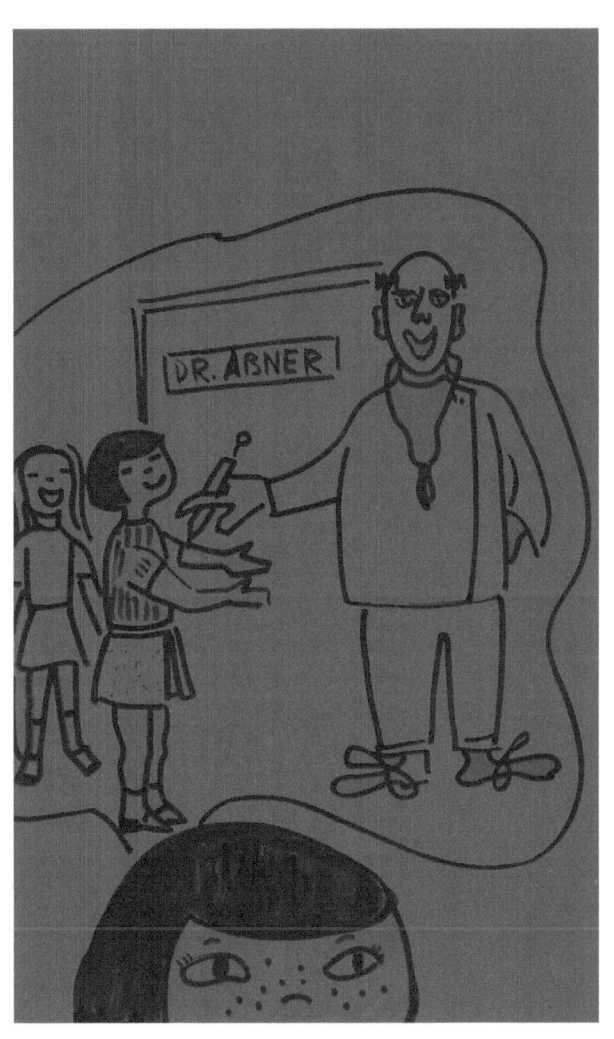

"AND AFTER WE GO
TO SEE DR. ADLER FOR
A WHILE, YOU WILL STOP
SNEEZING AND WHEEZING.
YOUR EYES WILL NOT GET
RED AND REDDER. AND
THE MONEY WE SAVE
FROM NOT USING
TRILLIONS
OF TISSUES WILL BUY YOU
A CAT OF YOUR VERY OWN!
THAT IS, JUST AS SOON
AS DR. ADLER PERMISTS IT!"

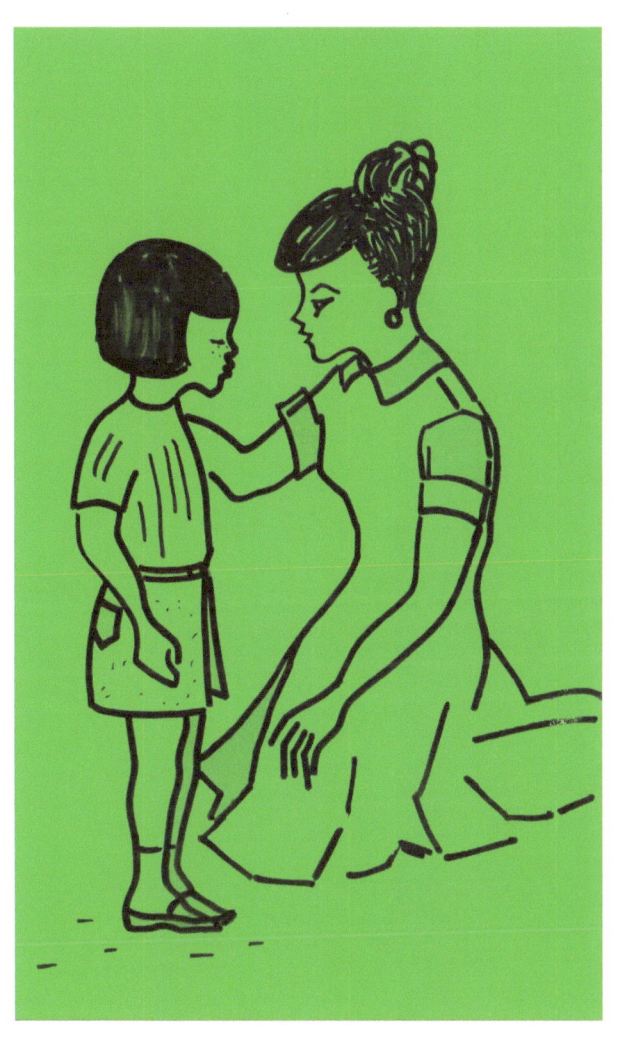

Betty Forhman is a writer and retired social work executive who lives in New York City.

Notes for Parents

Dates for Allergist's Visits

www.ingramcontent.com/pod-product-compliance
Lightning Source LLC
Chambersburg PA
CBHW040316010626
45792CB00022B/605